MW01231303

## This book is dedicated to...

My parents who have loved, nurtured & encouraged me.
Excellent doctors and nurses everywhere.
But especially, Dr. George Burke, Dr. Gaetano Ciancio and Dr. Robert Sonneborn.
Ultimately, Jehovah who makes anything possible.
With A Healthy Heart,
Love Carol

With love to my granddaughter, Tabitha Mae Stephens,
who is showing every sign of becoming an artist herself some day.
Love, Gramma 'Chelle

Library of Congress CIP 2004108309
ISBN 0-975888-0-5 $16.95

Editor: Carol Hamm
Illustration: Michelle Morse
Cover Design and Layout: Kelly Harris
Book Production: Print On Demand
Printed in Hong Kong
First Edition
Printed on partially recycled paper

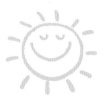

HiS SONSHINE INC.
PO BOX 6669
DELRAY BEACH, FL. 33482

A portion of the profit from this book will go directly to
The Transplant Foundation; and to help underprivileged children around the world.

# ABC'S
# FOR YOUR
# HEALTH

## By Carol Hamm

### illustrated by Michelle Morse

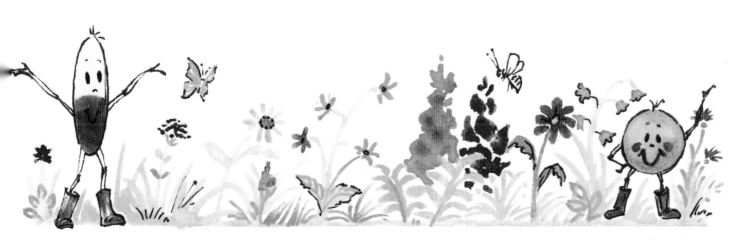

Look for the two of us on every page...

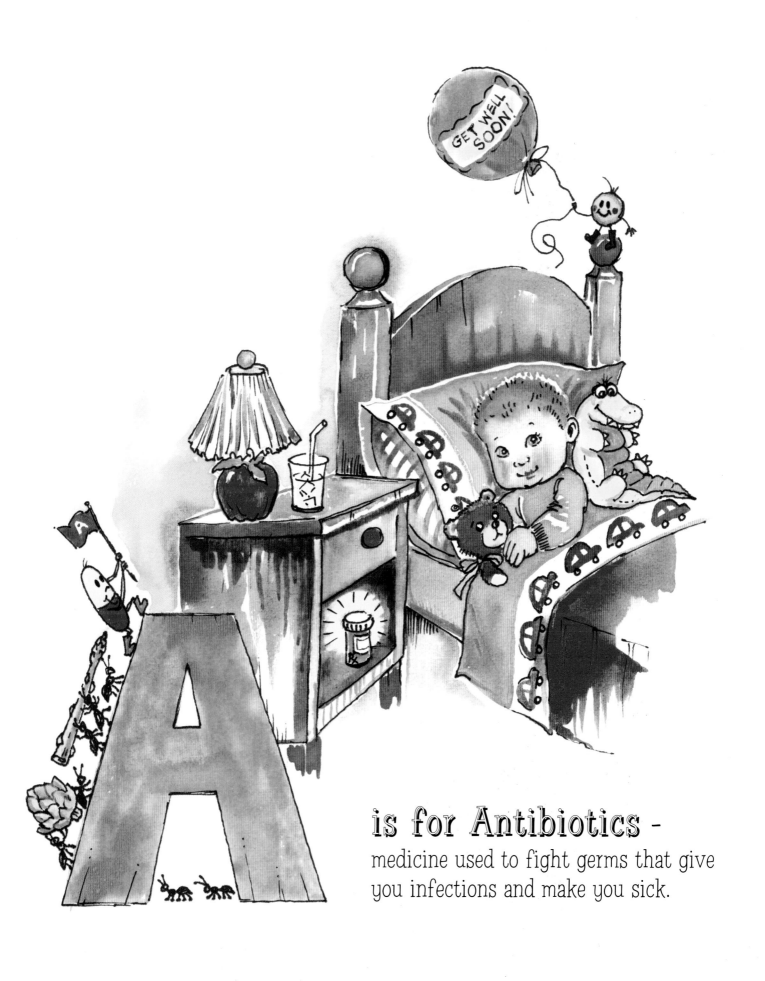

**is for Antibiotics -**
medicine used to fight germs that give
you infections and make you sick.

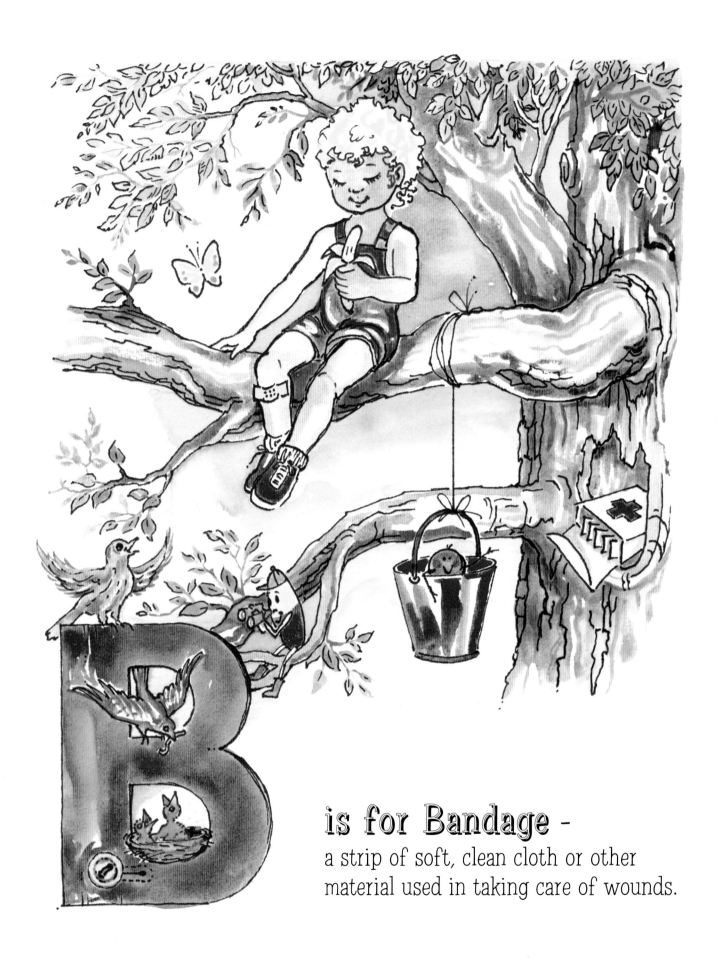

**is for Bandage -**
a strip of soft, clean cloth or other
material used in taking care of wounds.

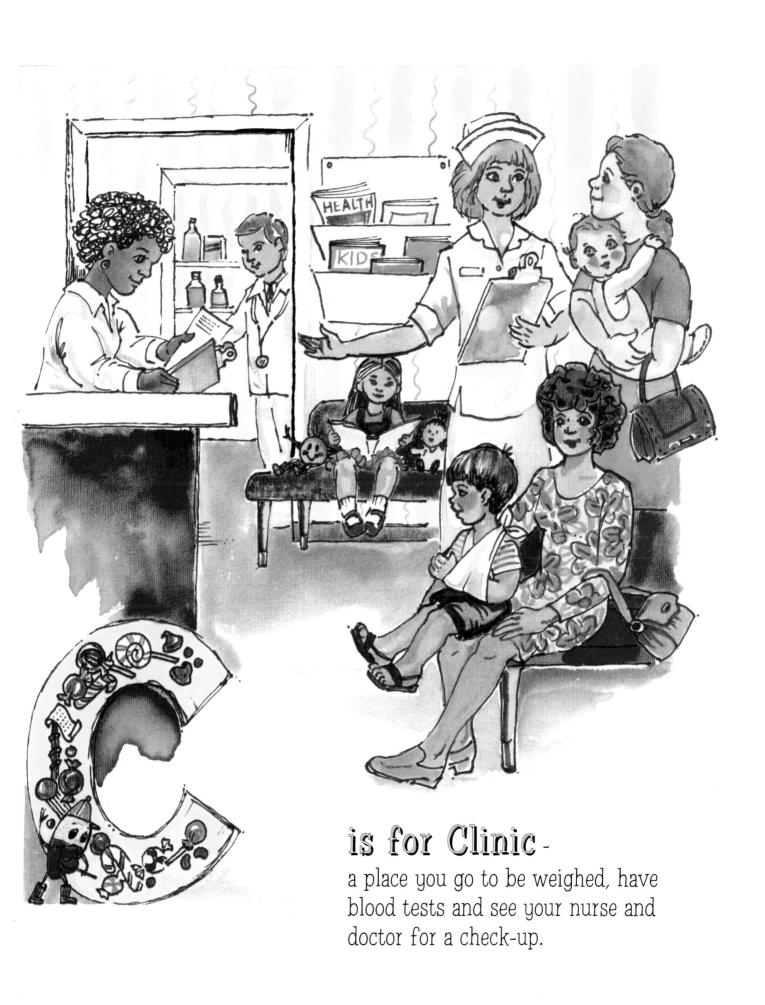

**is for Clinic** -
a place you go to be weighed, have
blood tests and see your nurse and
doctor for a check-up.

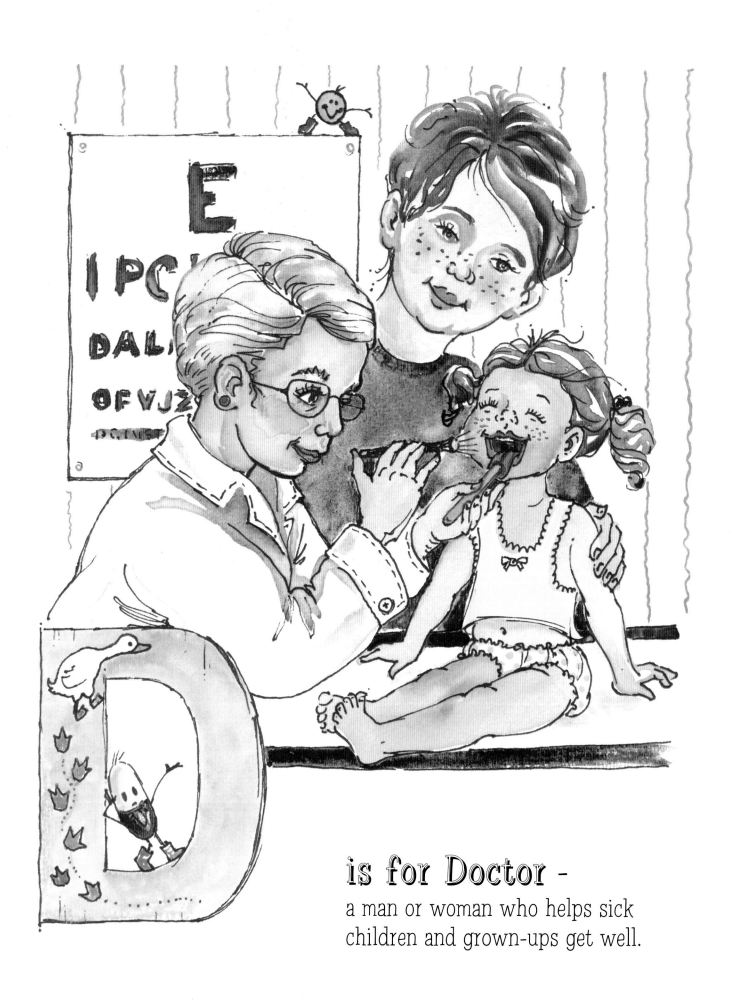

**is for Doctor -**
a man or woman who helps sick
children and grown-ups get well.

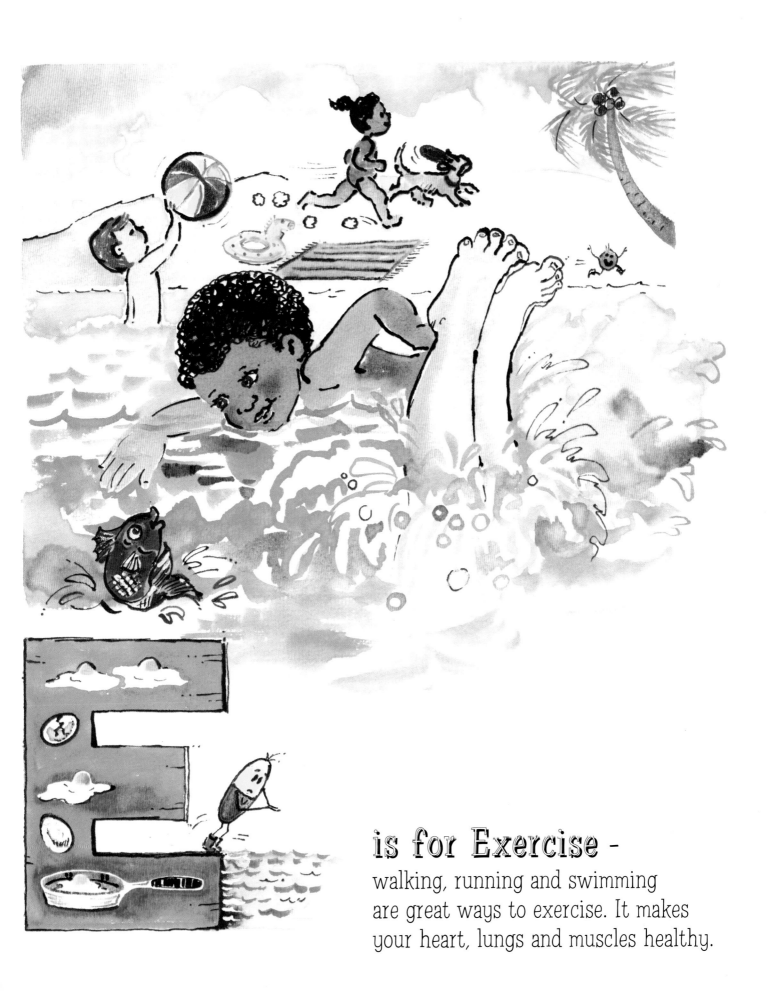

is for Exercise -
walking, running and swimming
are great ways to exercise. It makes
your heart, lungs and muscles healthy.

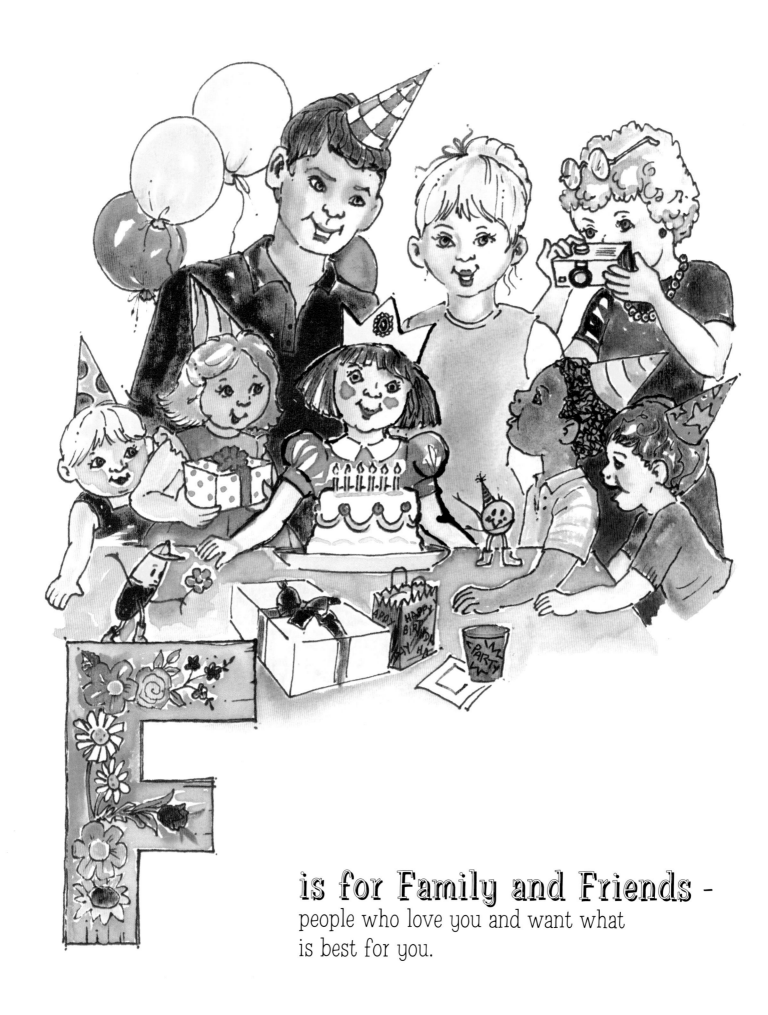

**is for Family and Friends -**
people who love you and want what
is best for you.

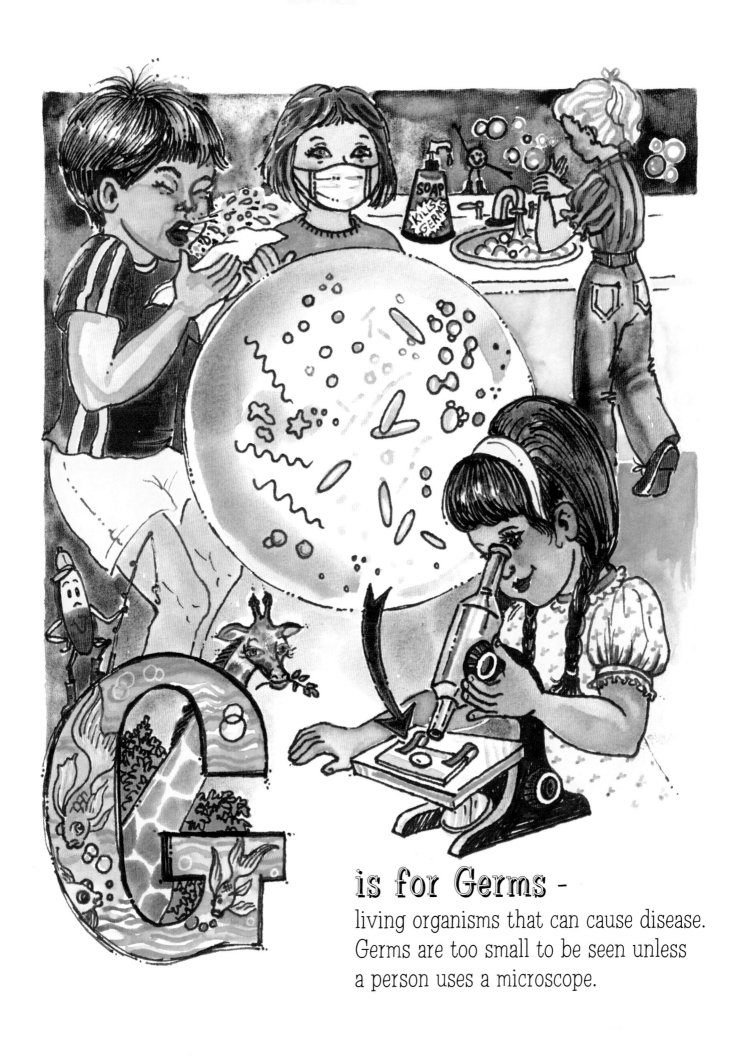

**is for Germs -**
living organisms that can cause disease.
Germs are too small to be seen unless
a person uses a microscope.

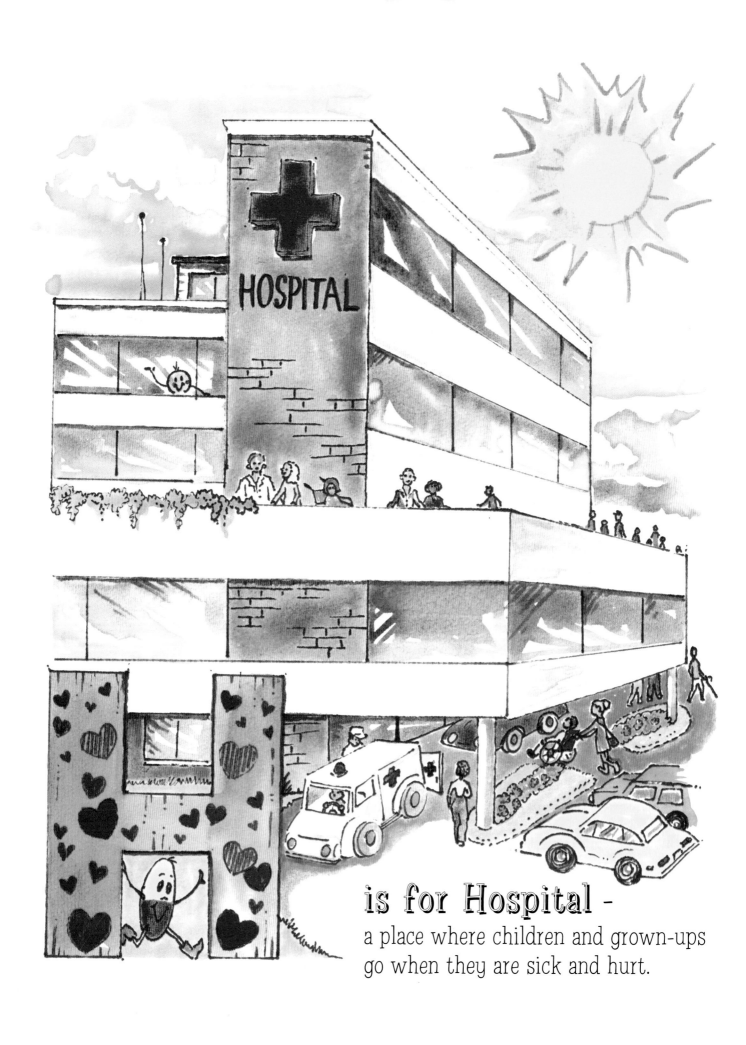

is for Hospital -
a place where children and grown-ups
go when they are sick and hurt.

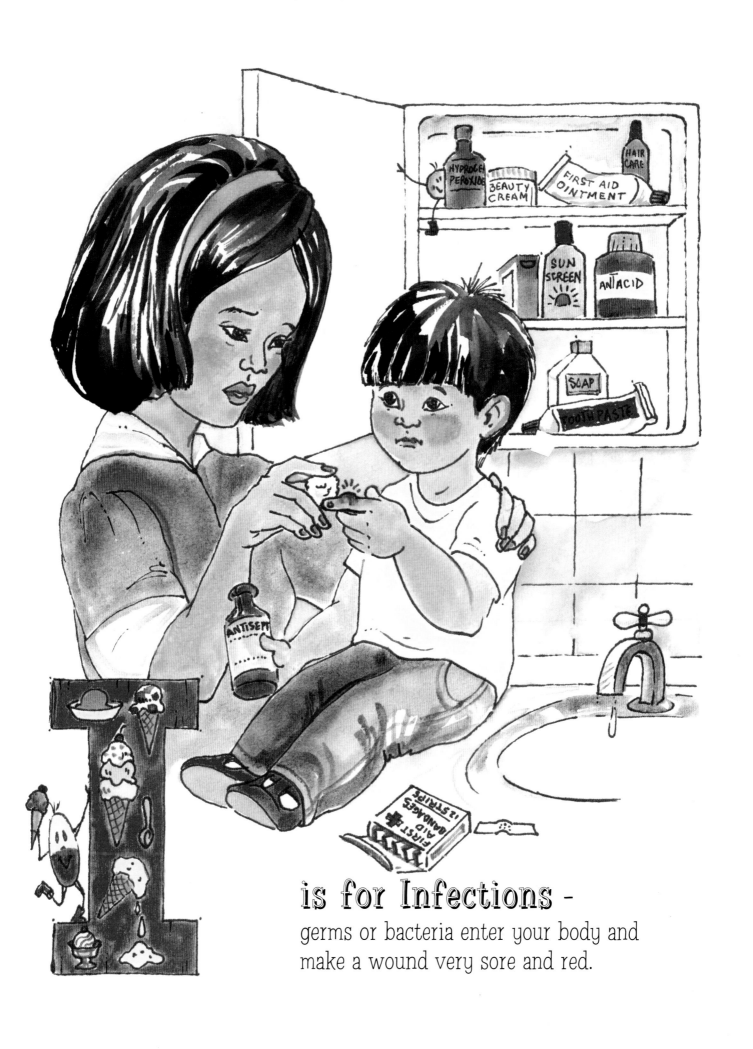

**is for Infections –**
germs or bacteria enter your body and
make a wound very sore and red.

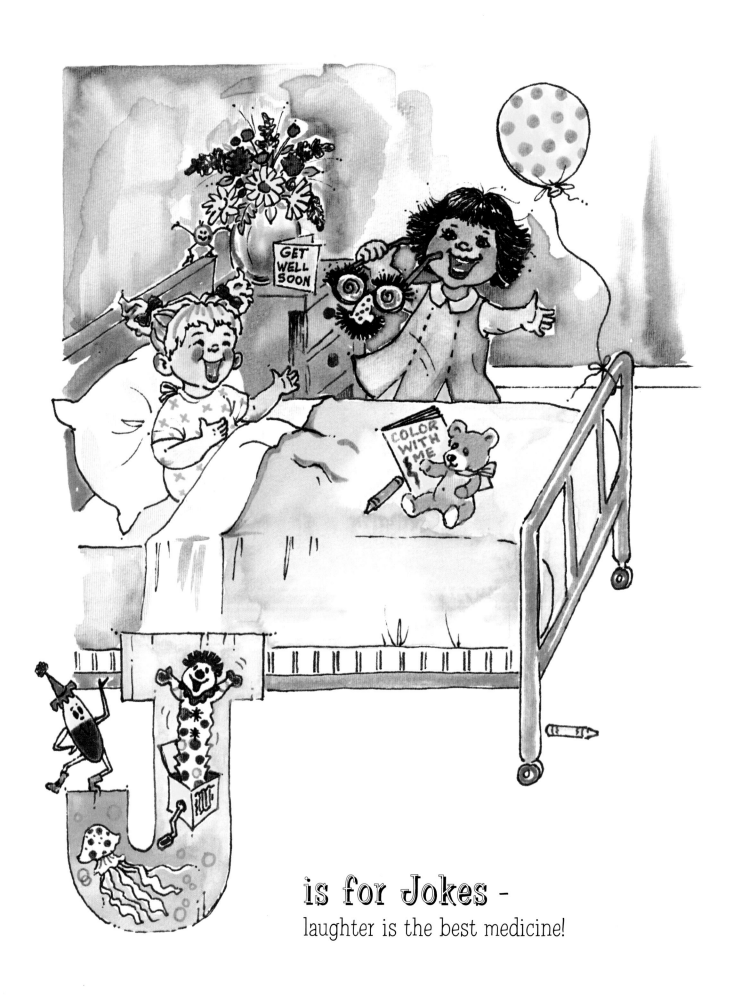

is for Jokes -
laughter is the best medicine!

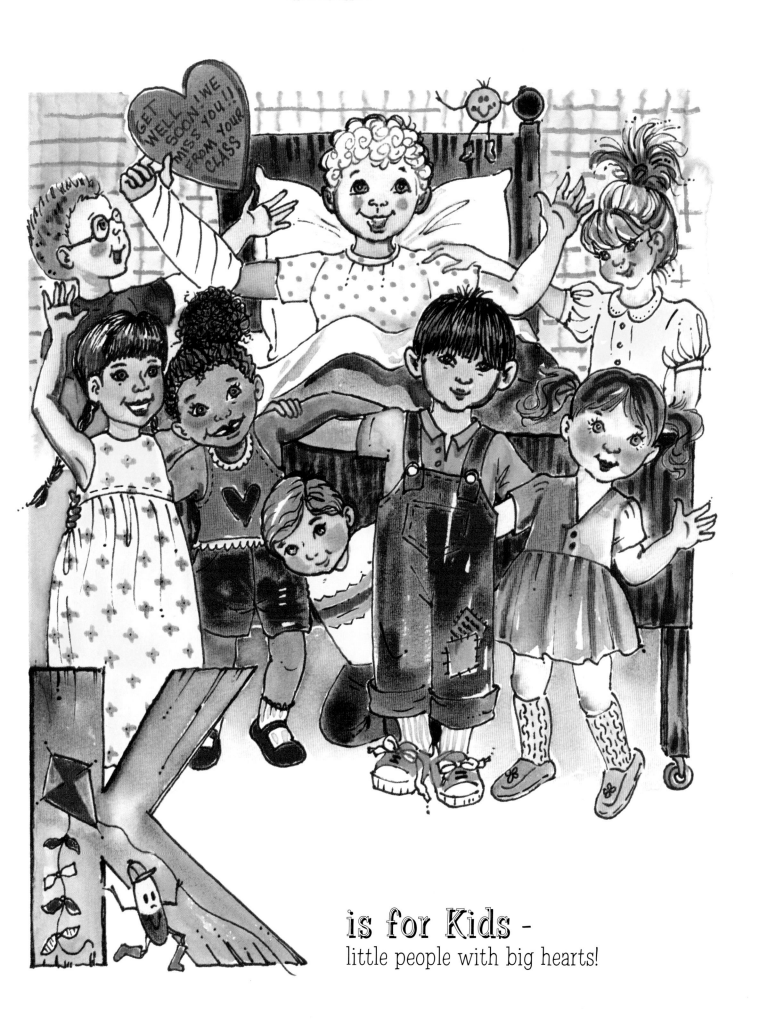

**is for Kids** -
little people with big hearts!

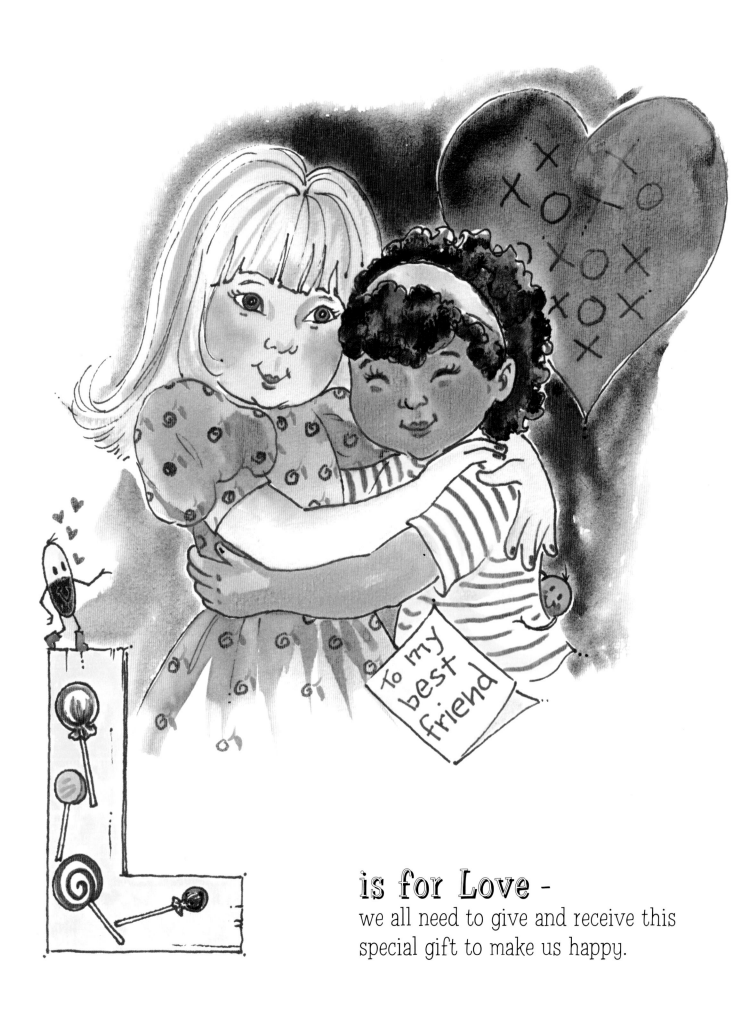

**is for Love -**
we all need to give and receive this
special gift to make us happy.

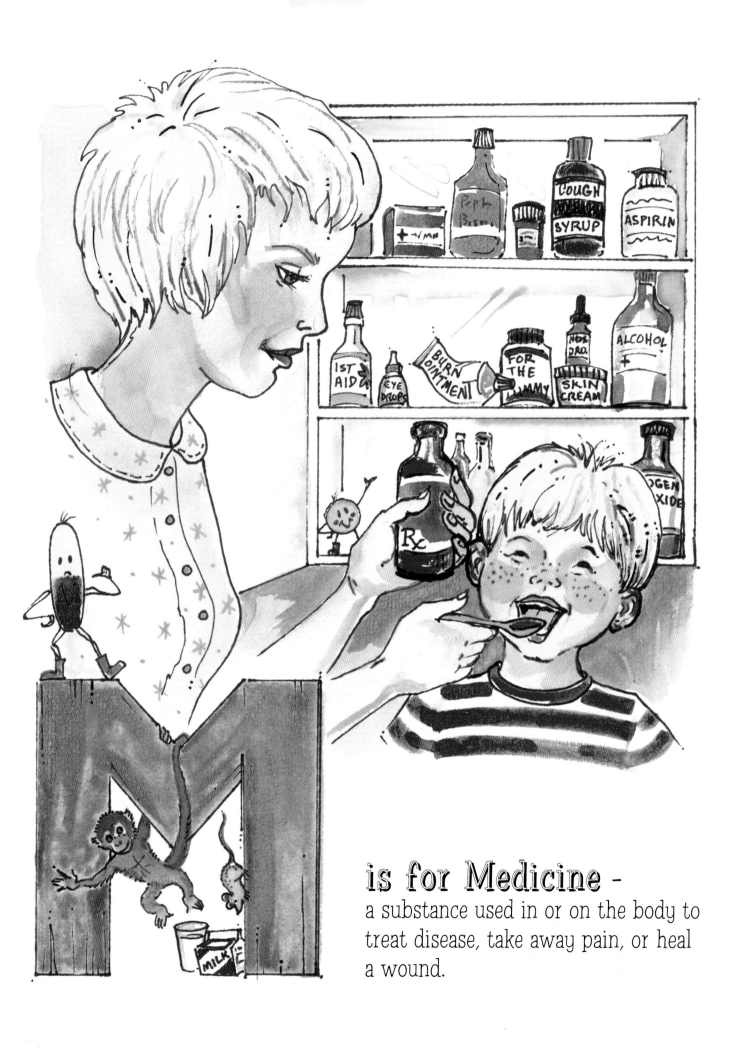

**is for Medicine** -
a substance used in or on the body to
treat disease, take away pain, or heal
a wound.

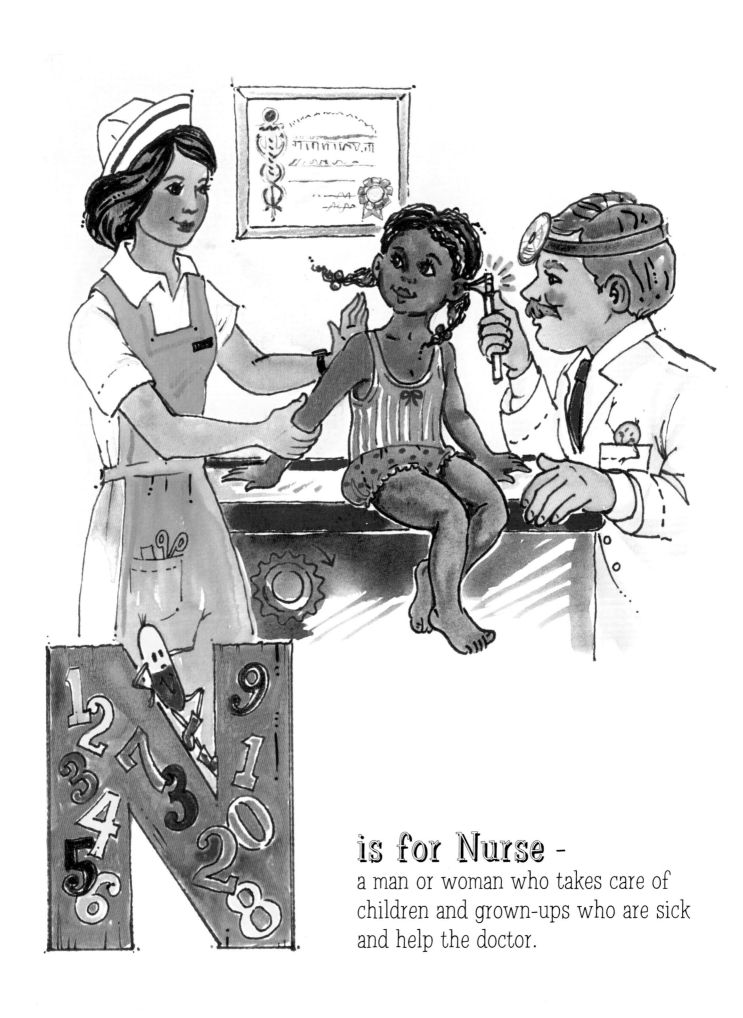

**is for Nurse -**
a man or woman who takes care of
children and grown-ups who are sick
and help the doctor.

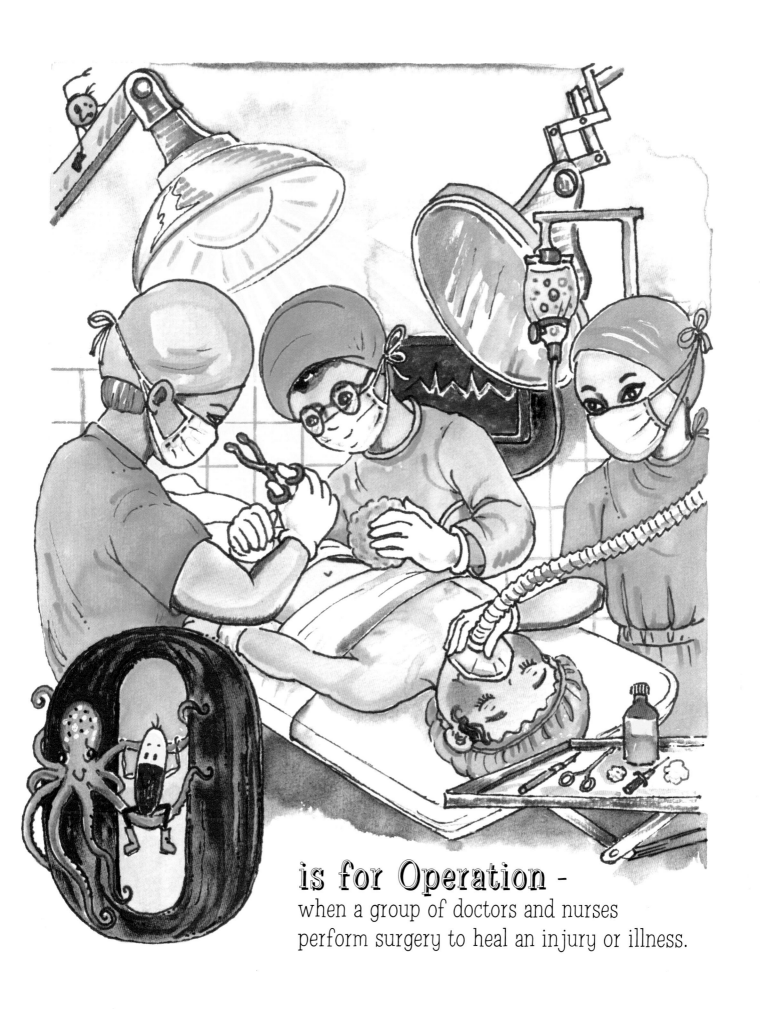

is for Operation -
when a group of doctors and nurses
perform surgery to heal an injury or illness.

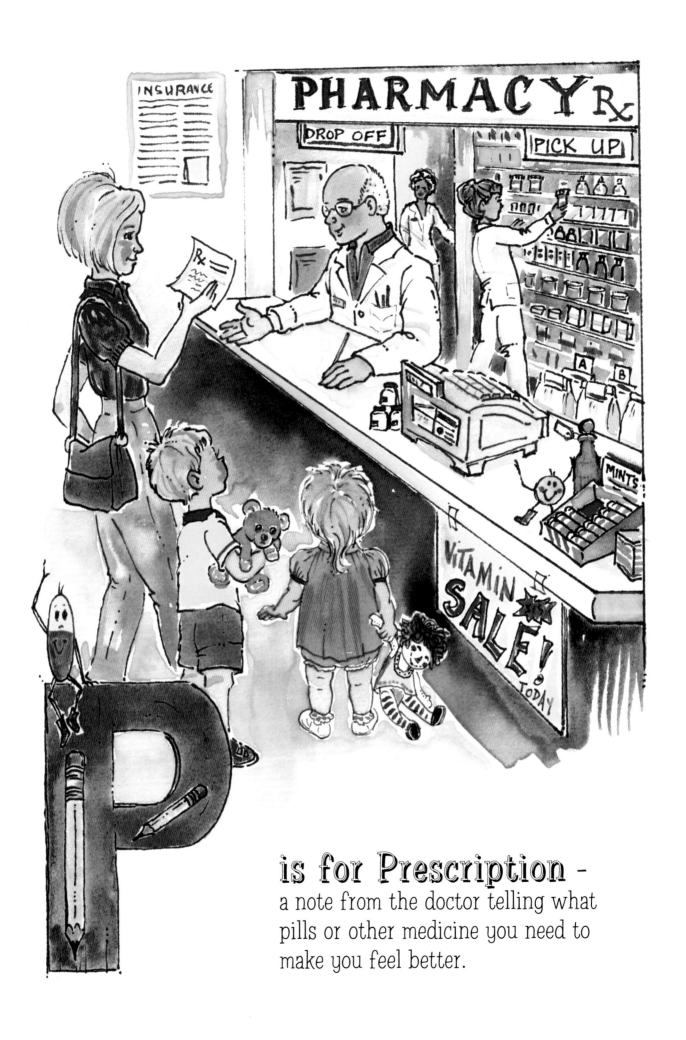

**is for Prescription** –
a note from the doctor telling what
pills or other medicine you need to
make you feel better.

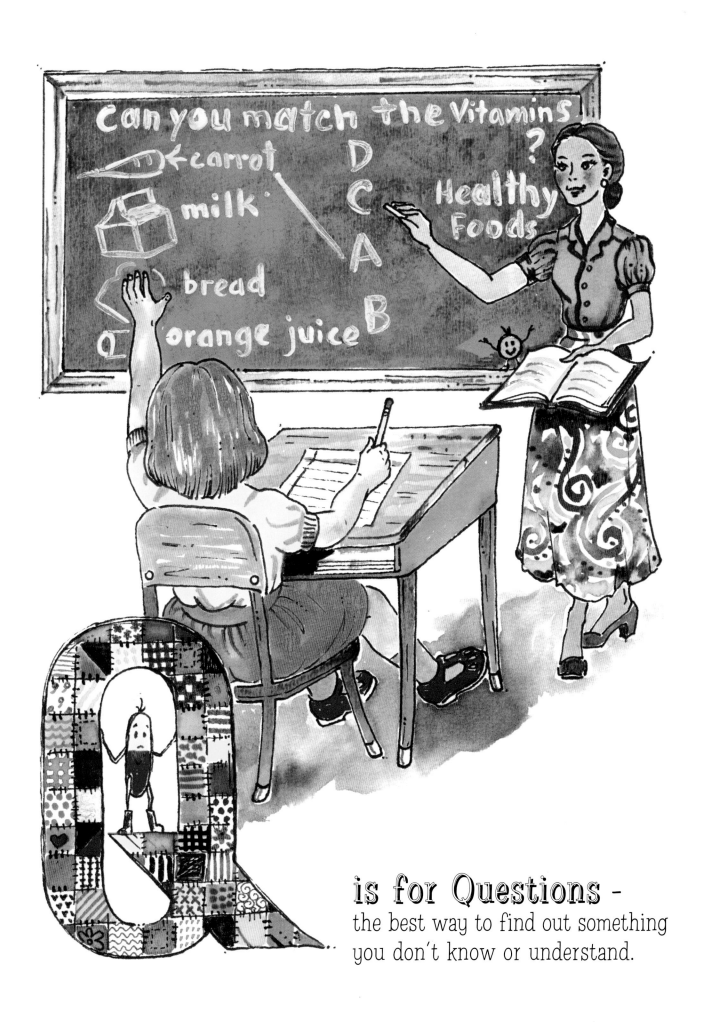

**is for Questions** –
the best way to find out something
you don't know or understand.

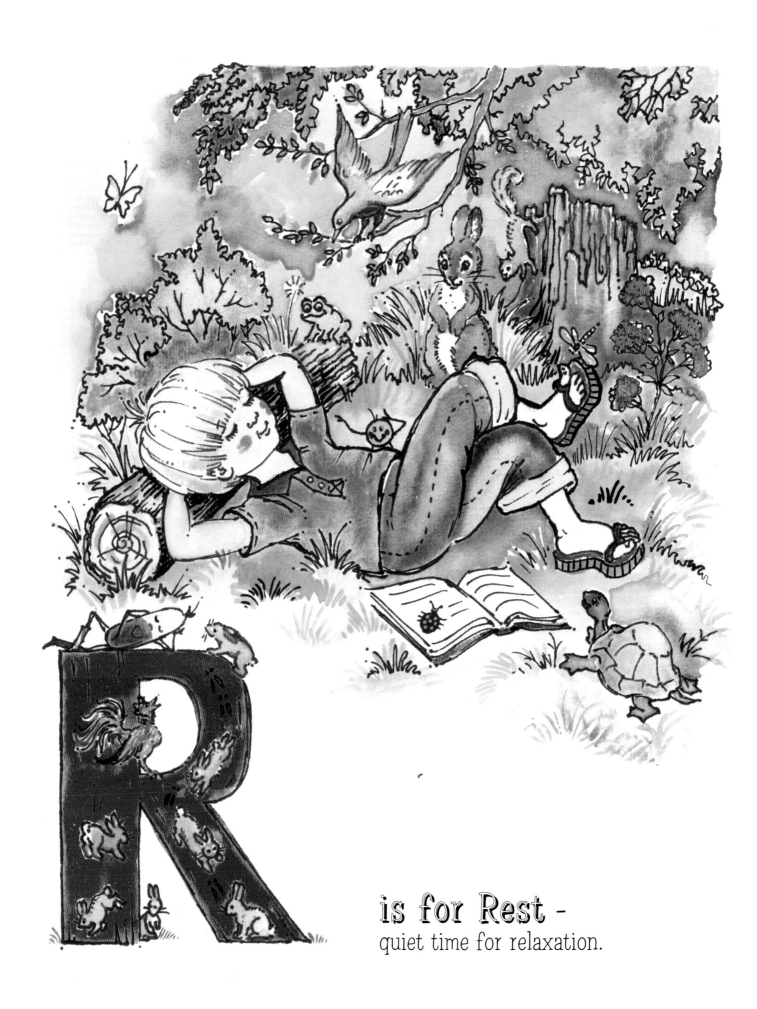

**is for Rest -**
quiet time for relaxation.

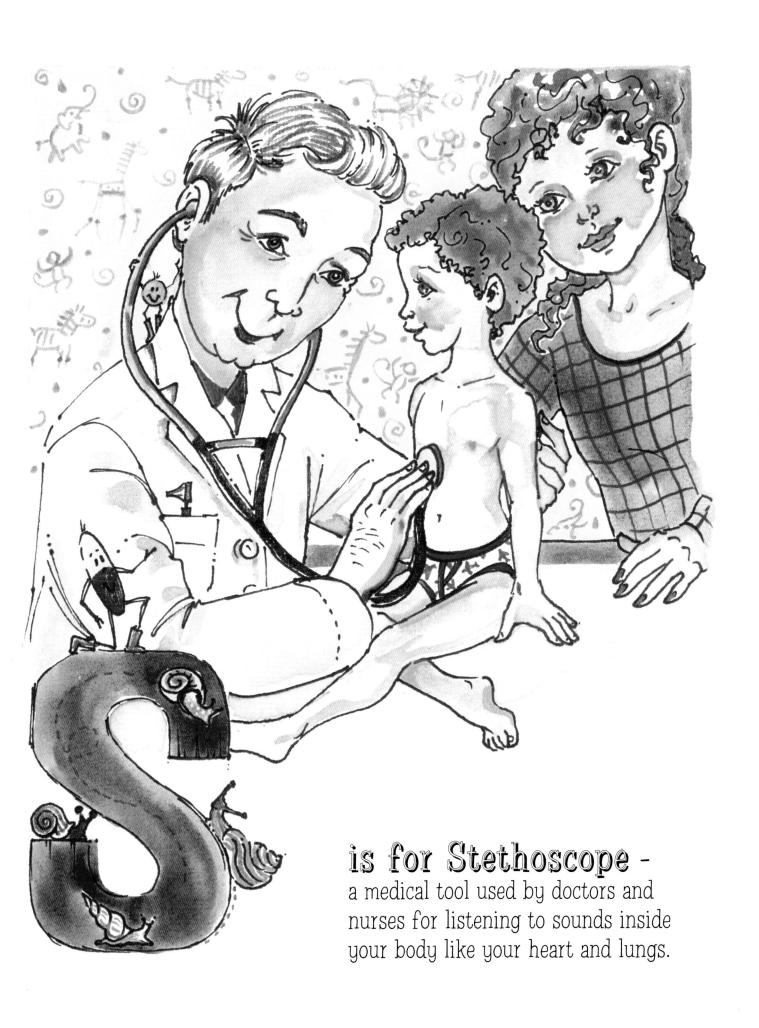

# is for Stethoscope -
a medical tool used by doctors and nurses for listening to sounds inside your body like your heart and lungs.

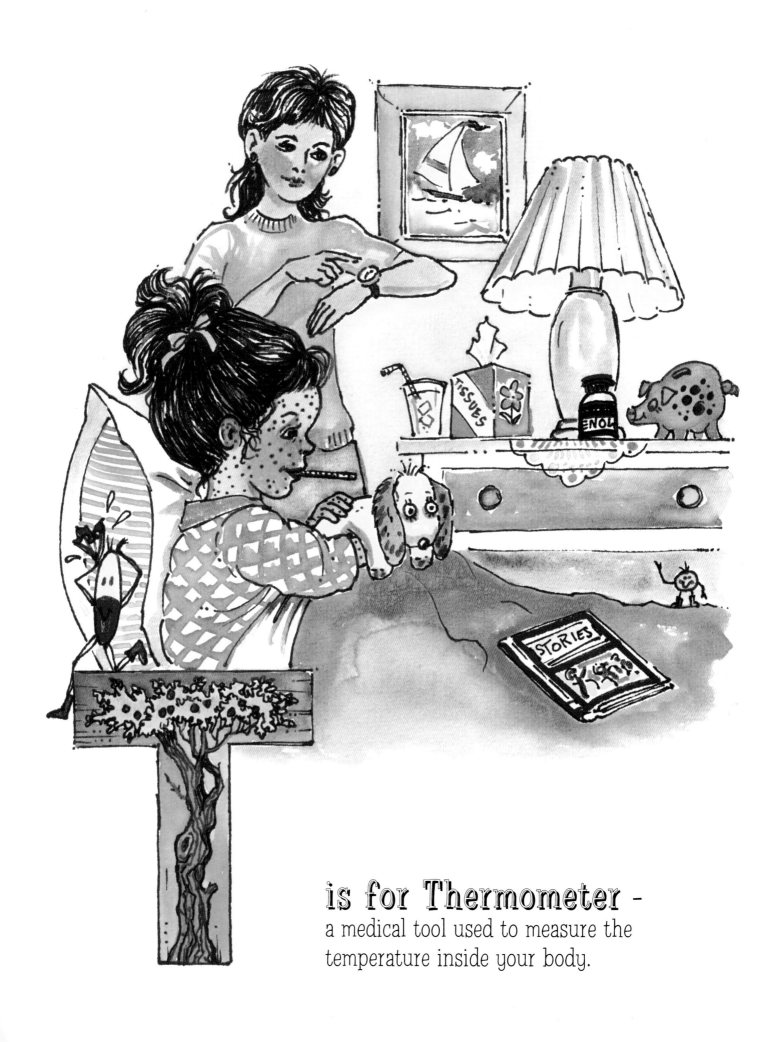

is for Thermometer -
a medical tool used to measure the
temperature inside your body.

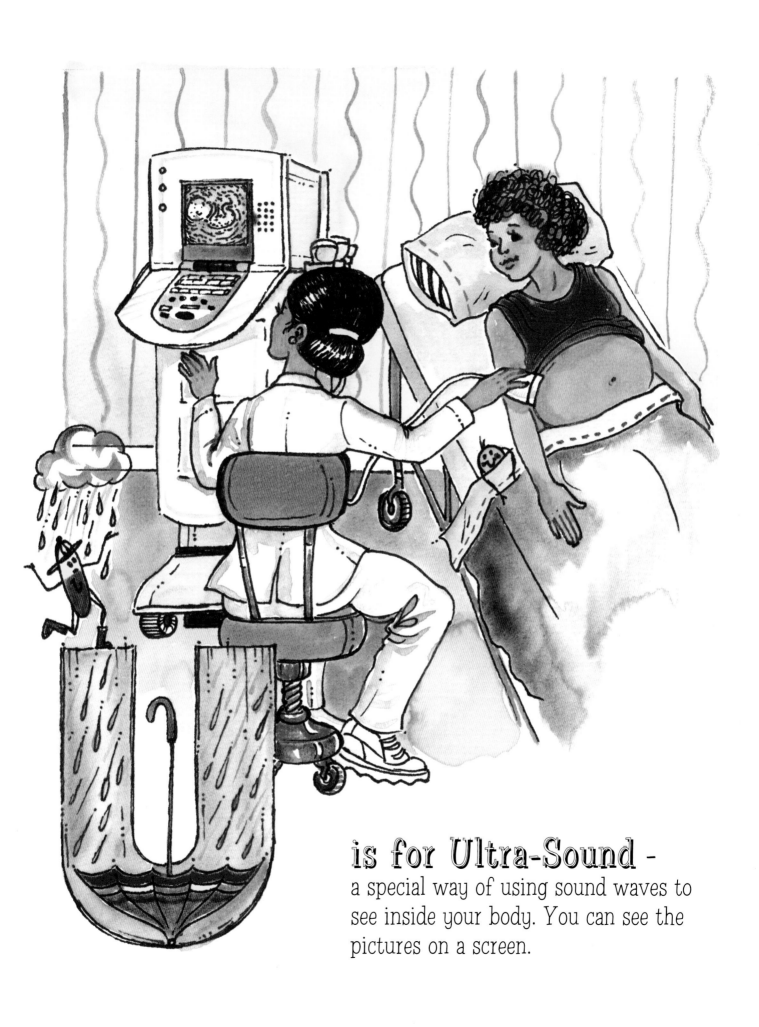

**is for Ultra-Sound** - a special way of using sound waves to see inside your body. You can see the pictures on a screen.

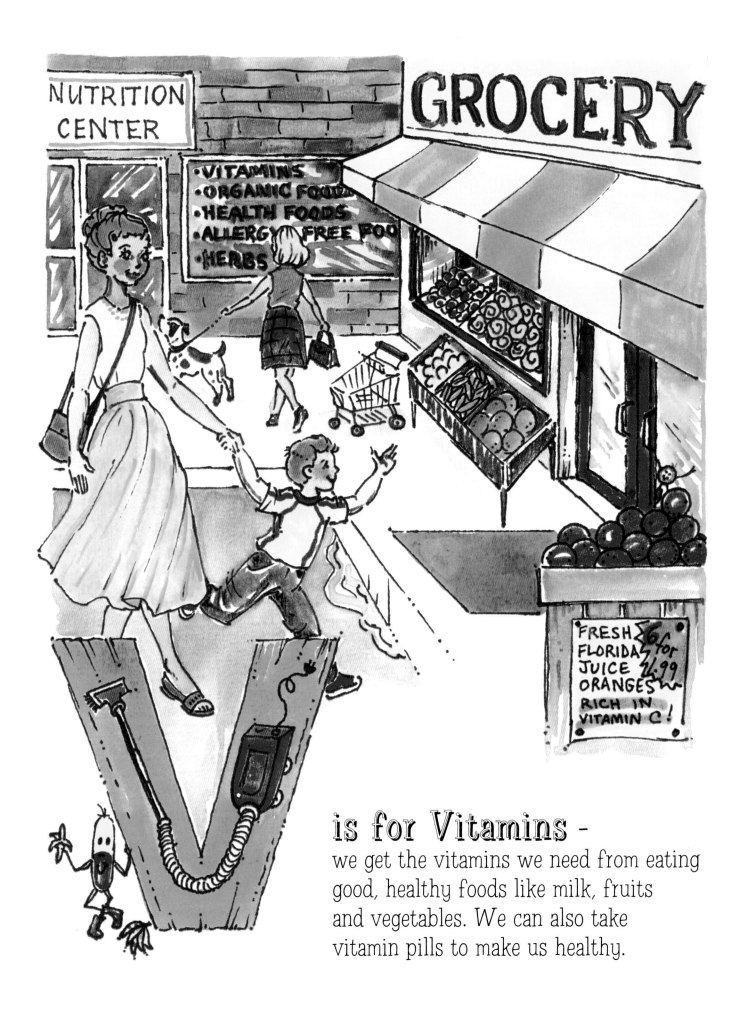

**is for Vitamins -**
we get the vitamins we need from eating
good, healthy foods like milk, fruits
and vegetables. We can also take
vitamin pills to make us healthy.

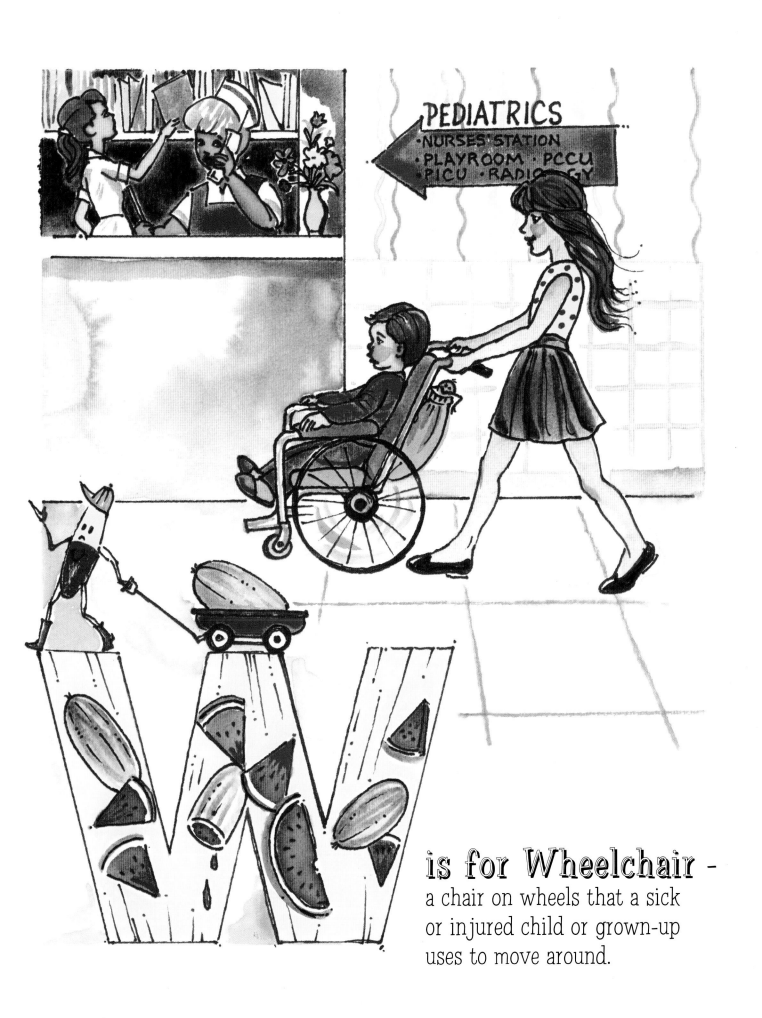

**is for Wheelchair** -
a chair on wheels that a sick
or injured child or grown-up
uses to move around.

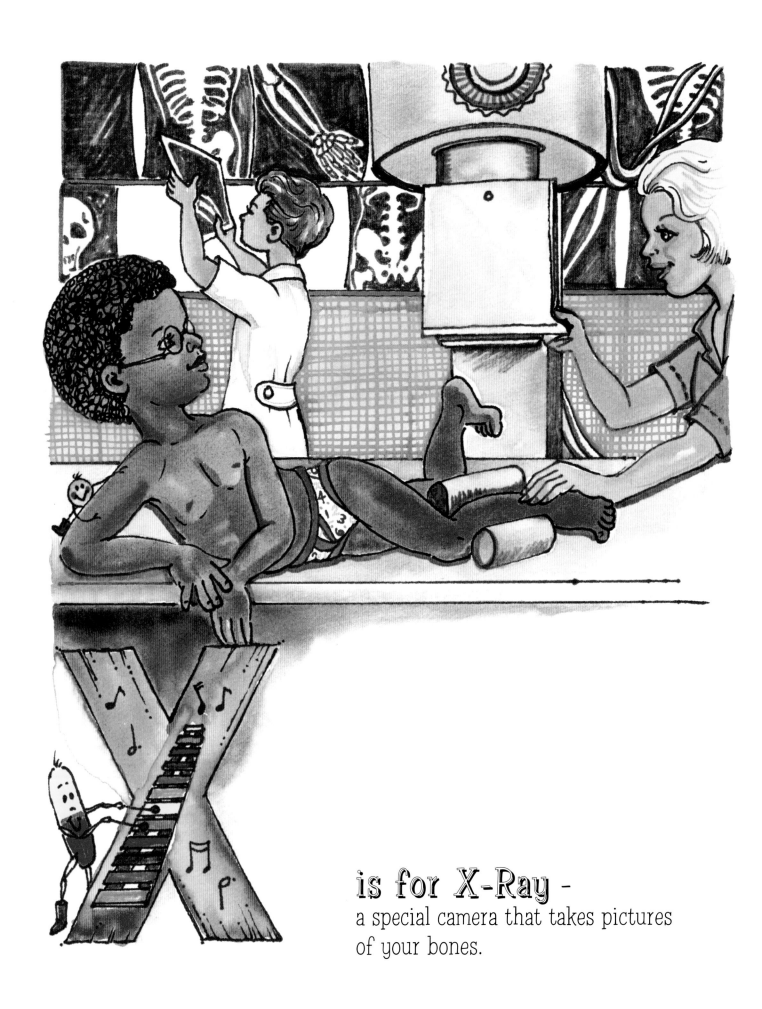

is for X-Ray -
a special camera that takes pictures
of your bones.

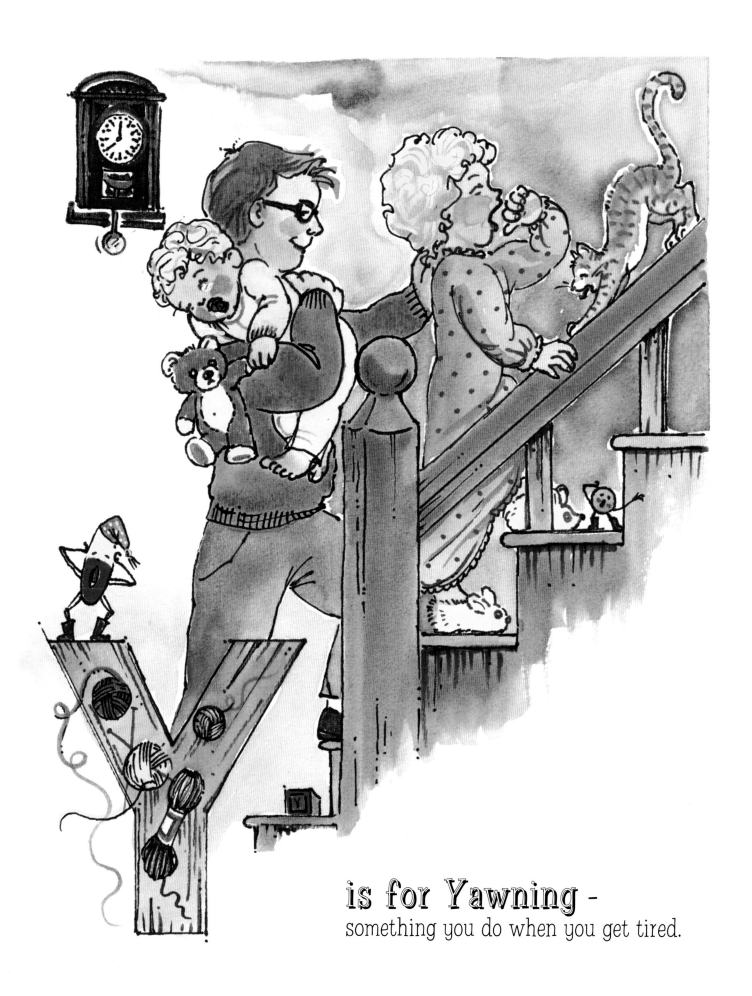

is for Yawning -
something you do when you get tired.

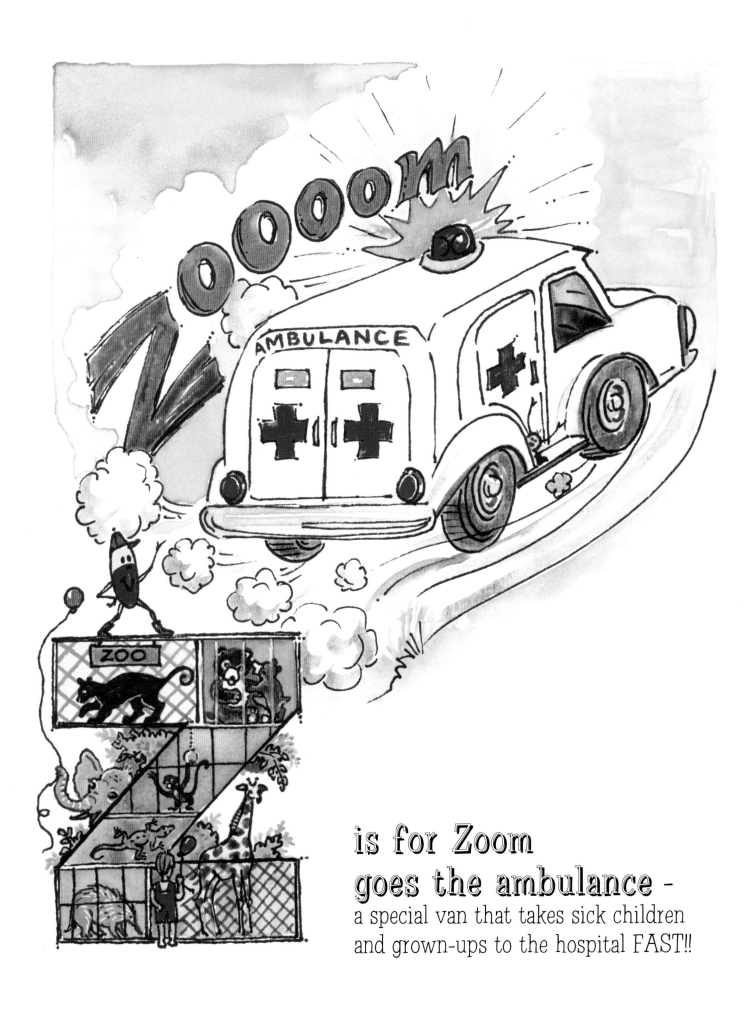

**is for Zoom
goes the ambulance -**
a special van that takes sick children
and grown-ups to the hospital FAST!!

Let's do a review
and see how you do.
Say the missing letter,
and you'll be feeling better!!!

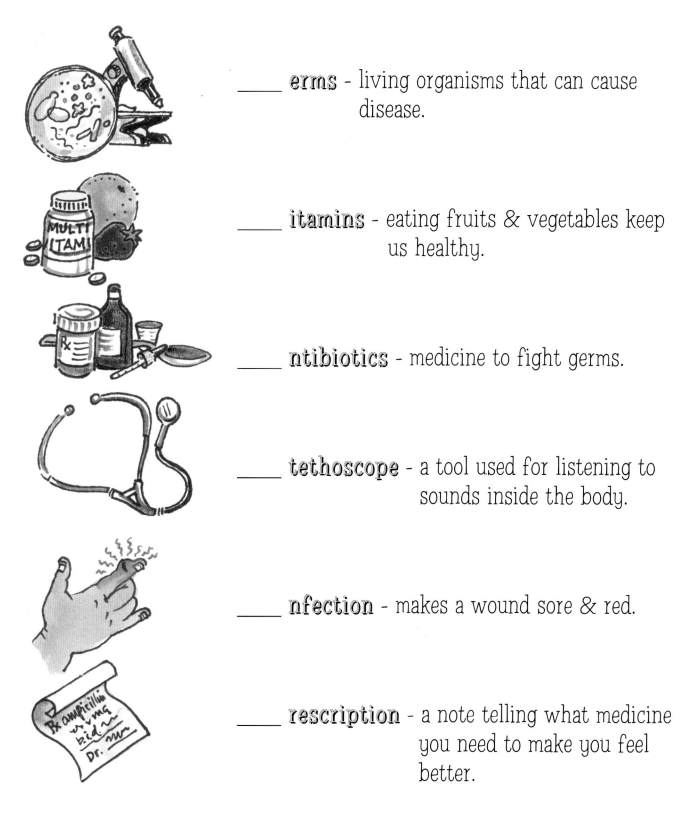

_____ erms - living organisms that can cause disease.

_____ itamins - eating fruits & vegetables keep us healthy.

_____ ntibiotics - medicine to fight germs.

_____ tethoscope - a tool used for listening to sounds inside the body.

_____ nfection - makes a wound sore & red.

_____ rescription - a note telling what medicine you need to make you feel better.

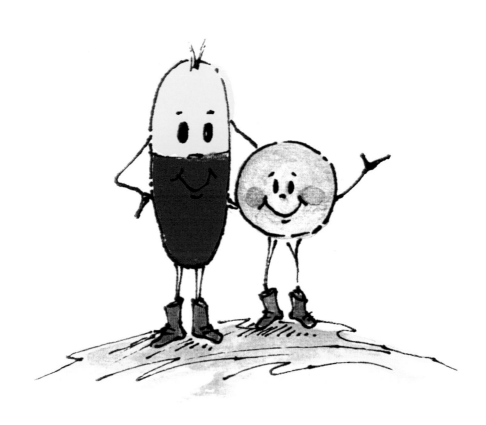